The Greatest Plant Based Diet Cooking Guide

Innovative Ways for Healthier Meals

Jason Noel

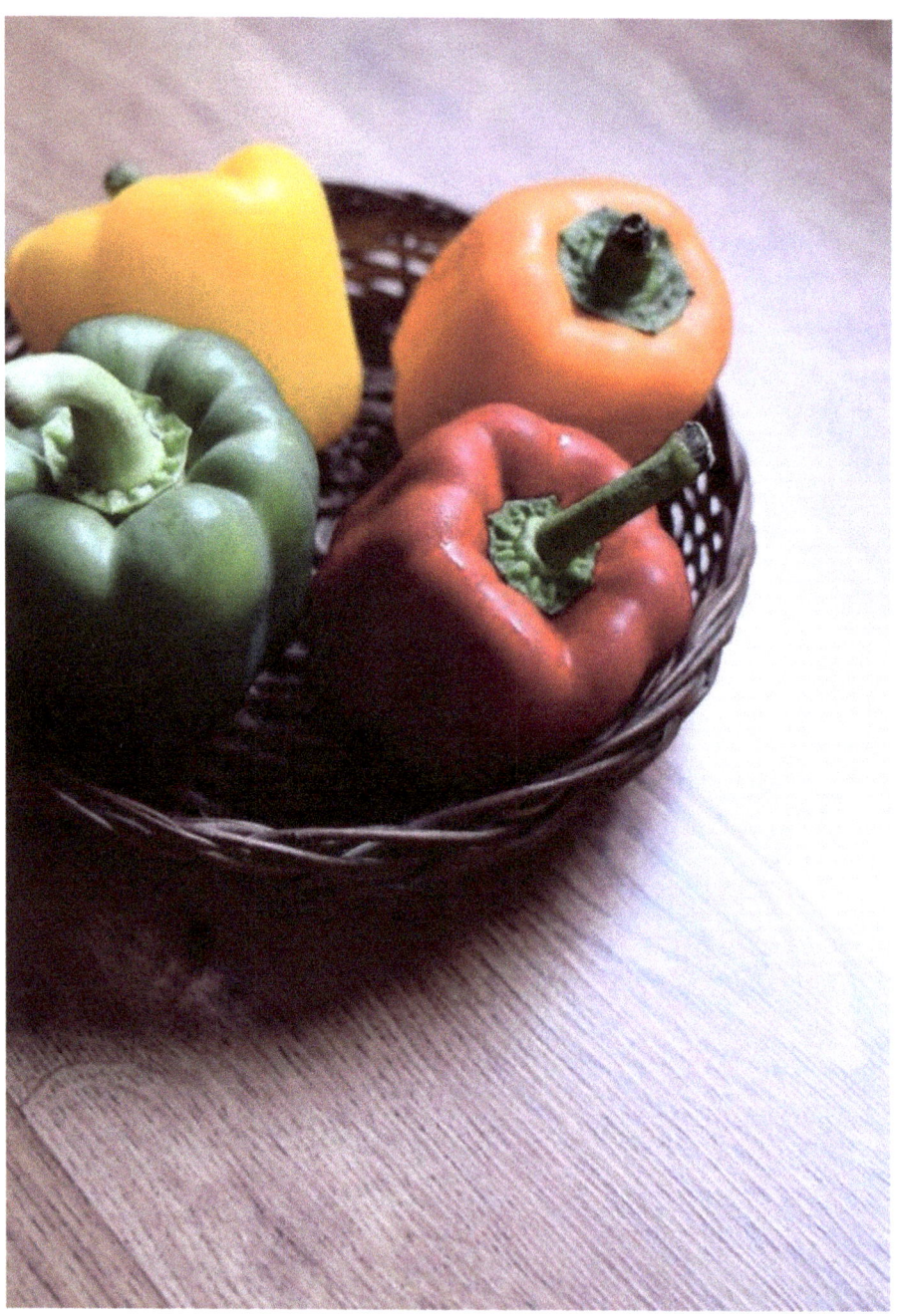

Table of Contents

Mixed Seed Crackers

Preparation Time: 15-30 minutes | Cooking Time: 50 minutes | Servings: 4

Ingredients:

- ⅓ cup coconut flour

- ⅓ cup sesame seeds

- ⅓ cup sunflower seeds

- ⅓ cup chia seeds

- ⅓ cup pumpkin seeds

- 1 tsp salt

- ¼ cup plant butter, melted

- 1 cup boiling water

Directions:

- Preheat an oven to 300 F and line a baking sheet with parchment paper.

- In a medium bowl, mix the coconut flour, sesame seeds, sunflower seeds, chia seeds, pumpkin seeds, and salt.

• Add the plant butter, boiling water, and mix until well combined.

• Spread the mixture on the baking sheet and bake in the oven for 45 minutes until the crackers are firm.

• Remove the crackers and allow cooling for 10 minutes.

• Break the crackers into pieces and enjoy!

Nutrition:

Calories 725 | Fats 67. 2g | Carbs 18. 1g | Protein 24. 3g

Seitan Bell Pepper Balls

Preparation Time: 15-30 minutes | Cooking Time: 25 minutes | Servings: 4

Ingredients:

• 1 tbsp flax seed powder + 3 tbsp water

• 1 lb seitan, crumbled

• ¼ cup chopped mixed bell peppers

• Salt and black pepper to taste

• 1 tbsp almond flour

• 1 tsp garlic powder

• 1 tsp onion powder

• 1 tsp tofu mayonnaise

• Olive oil for brushing

Directions:

• Preheat the oven to 400 F and line a baking sheet with parchment paper.

• In a medium bowl, mix the flax seed powder with water and allow thickening for 5 minutes.

• Add the seitan, bell peppers, salt, black pepper, almond flour, garlic powder, onion powder, and tofu mayonnaise. Mix well and form 1-inch balls from the mixture.

• Arrange on the baking sheet, brush with cooking spray, and bake in the oven for 15 to 20 minutes or until brown and compacted.

• Remove from the oven and serve.

Nutrition:

Calories 492 | Fats 41. 3g | Carbs 4. 1g | Protein 26. 5g

Quinoa Stuffed Tomatoes

Preparation Time: 15-30 minutes | Cooking Time: 50 minutes | Servings: 4

Ingredients:

• 8 medium-sized tomatoes

• ¾ cup quinoa, rinsed and drained

• 1 ½ cups water

• 1 tbsp olive oil

• 1 small onion, diced

• 3 garlic cloves, minced

• Salt and black pepper to taste

• 1 cup chopped spinach

• 1 (7 oz) can chickpeas, drained and rinsed

• ½ cup chopped fresh basil

Directions:

• Preheat the oven to 400 F.

• Cut off the heads of tomatoes and use a paring knife to scoop the inner pulp of the tomatoes. Season with some olive oil, salt, and black pepper.

• Add the quinoa and water to a medium pot, season with salt, and cook for 10 to 15 minutes until the quinoa is tender and the water is absorbed. Fluff and set aside.

• Heat the remaining olive oil in a medium skillet and sauté the onion and garlic until softened and fragrant, 30 seconds.

• Mix in the spinach and cook until wilted, 2 minutes. Stir in the basil, chickpeas, and quinoa; allow warming from 2 minutes.

• Spoon the mixture into the tomatoes, place the tomatoes into the baking dish and bake in the oven for 20 minutes or until the tomatoes soften. Remove the tomatoes from the oven and dish the food. Serve warm.

Nutrition:

Calories 296 kcal | Fats 7. 5g | Carbs 48. 3g | Protein 12g

Cajun Sweet Potato Chips

Preparation Time: 15-30 minutes | Cooking Time: 55 minutes | Servings: 4

Ingredients:

• 2 sweet potatoes, peeled and thinly sliced

• Salt to season

• 2 tbsp melted plant butter

• 1 tbsp Cajun seasoning

Directions:

• Preheat the oven to 400 F and line a baking sheet with parchment paper.

• In a medium bowl, add the sweet potatoes, salt, plant butter, and Cajun seasoning. Toss well. Spread the chips on the baking sheet making sure not to overlap and bake in the oven for 50 minutes to 1 hour or until crispy.

• Remove the sheet and pour the chips into a large bowl.

• Allow cooling and enjoy.

Nutrition:

• Calories 65 | Fats 5. 9g | Carbs 2. 8g | Protein 1g

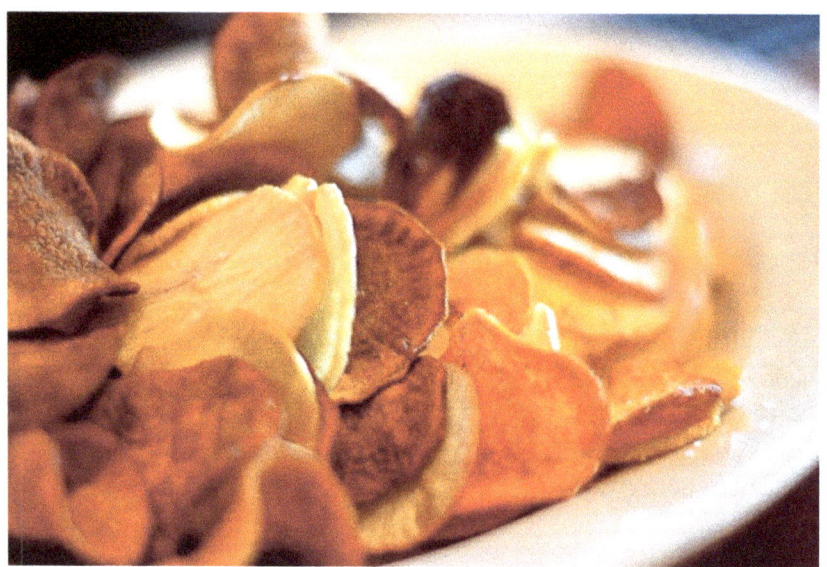

Maple Cinnamon Popcorn

Preparation Time: 15-30 minutes | Cooking Time: 15 minutes | Servings: 4

Ingredients:

- ½ cup popcorn kernels

- ¼ tsp cinnamon powder

- ½ tsp pure maple syrup

- 1 tsp plant butter, melted

- Salt to taste

Directions:

• Pour the popcorn kernels into a large pot and set over medium heat. Cover the lid and allow the kernels to pop completely. Shake the pot a few times to ensure even popping, 10 minutes.

• Meanwhile, in a small bowl, mix the cinnamon powder, maple syrup, butter, and salt. When the popcorn is ready, turn the heat off, and toss in the cinnamon mixture until well distributed. Pour the popcorn into serving bowls, allow cooling, and enjoy.

Nutrition:

Calories 15 | Fats 1g | Carbs 1. 5g | Protein 0. 2g

Skewers of Mozzarella and Tomato

Preparation Time: 15 minutes | Cooking Time: 0 minutes | Servings: 8

Ingredients:

• 1 teaspoon pesto

• 250 g cherry tomatoes

• 250 g vegan mozzarella

• 1 bunch of basil

• 3 tablespoon olive oil

Directions:

• Wash and prepare the tomatoes.

• Pluck the basil leaves, cut the mozzarella into small cubes.

• Mix the pesto with the olive oil in a small bowl.

• Prepare wooden skewers and place two tomatoes, two basil leaves, and two cubes of mozzarella alternately on the skewers.

• Brush with a little pesto to serve.

Nutrition:

Calories: 259 | Fat: 15.4g | Carbs: 20.5g | Protein: 12.1g | Fiber: 3.2g

Filled Mushrooms

Preparation Time: 55 minutes | Cooking Time: 0 minutes | Servings: 2

Ingredients:

• 30 g pine nuts

• ½ lime

• ½ bunch of basil

• 8 large mushrooms

• 50 ml of water

• 115 g cashew nuts

• 2 tablespoon coconut milk

• Salt and pepper

Directions:

• Soak the cashew nuts in water the evening before.

• The drain water and fill the cores together with the basil, the coconut milk, the water, and the lime juice in a food processor.

• Process into a creamy puree.

• Clean the mushrooms and brush with the filling.

• Then bake in the oven at 180 degrees Celsius for about 15 minutes.

• In the meantime, toast the pine nuts in a small non-stick pan.

• Sprinkle the pine nuts over the mushrooms to serve.

Nutrition:

Calories: 239 | Fat: 11.4g | Carbs: 10.5g | Protein: 11.1g | Fiber: 3.2g

Pizza Bites

Preparation Time: 95 minutes | Cooking Time: 0 minutes | Servings: 8

Ingredients:

• 200 g flour

• 1 teaspoon salt

• 180 ml of water

• ½ cubes of yeast

• 1 teaspoon of sugar

• 250 g vegan salami

• 250 g vegan Gouda

Directions:

• Mix sugar, flour, and salt in a bowl.

• Make a well and crumble the yeast into it. Warm the water slightly and gradually pour it into the hollow.

• Mix the yeast and let it rise briefly, then work all the Ingredients in the bowl into a smooth dough.

- Let rise for 50 minutes, then roll out.

- Cut the cheese and salami into thin slices.

- Cut rectangles from the dough and cover the lower edge with cheese and salami. Roll up a little, cover again, and close the dough.

- Bake at 240 degrees Celsius for 10 to 12 minutes.

Nutrition:

- Calories: 289 | Fat: 15.4g | Carbs: 20.5g | Protein: 12.1g | Fiber: 3.2g

Filled Dough Pieces in Carrot Shape

Preparation Time: 30 minutes | Cooking Time: 0 minutes | Servings: 8

Ingredients:

• 400 ml vegetable stock

• 200 g red lentils

• 1 tablespoon almond butter

• 1 pack. Pizza dough

• salt and pepper

• 1 bunch of parsley

Directions:

• Do not make funnels out of aluminum paper to hold the pizza dough in the shape of a carrot.

• Roll out the dough, cut into strips and wrap around the funnels.

• Then bake at 200 degrees Celsius for about 10 minutes until they are golden brown.

• In the meantime, bring the broth to a boil and cook the lentils in it.

• Season with almond butter, salt, and pepper and let cool slightly.

• Fill the funnels with lentils and finally put a bunch of parsley on top.

• These bites go perfectly with an Easter brunch.

Nutrition:

Calories: 229 | Fat: 9.4g | Carbs: 11.5g | Protein: 12.1g | Fiber: 3.2g

Banana Cream Stuffed Strawberries

Preparation Time: 15-30 minutes | Cooking Time: 10 minutes | Servings: 4

Ingredients:

• 12 fresh strawberries, heads removed

• ¼ cup cashew cream

• ¼ tsp banana extract

• 1 tbsp unsweetened coconut flakes

Directions:

• Use a teaspoon to scoop out some of the strawberries pulp to create a hole within.

• In a small bowl, mix the cashew cream, banana extract, and maple syrup.

• Spoon the mixture into the strawberries and garnish with the coconut flakes. Serve.

Nutrition:

Calories 47 | Fats 3. 38g | Carbs 4. 11g | Protein 0. 69g

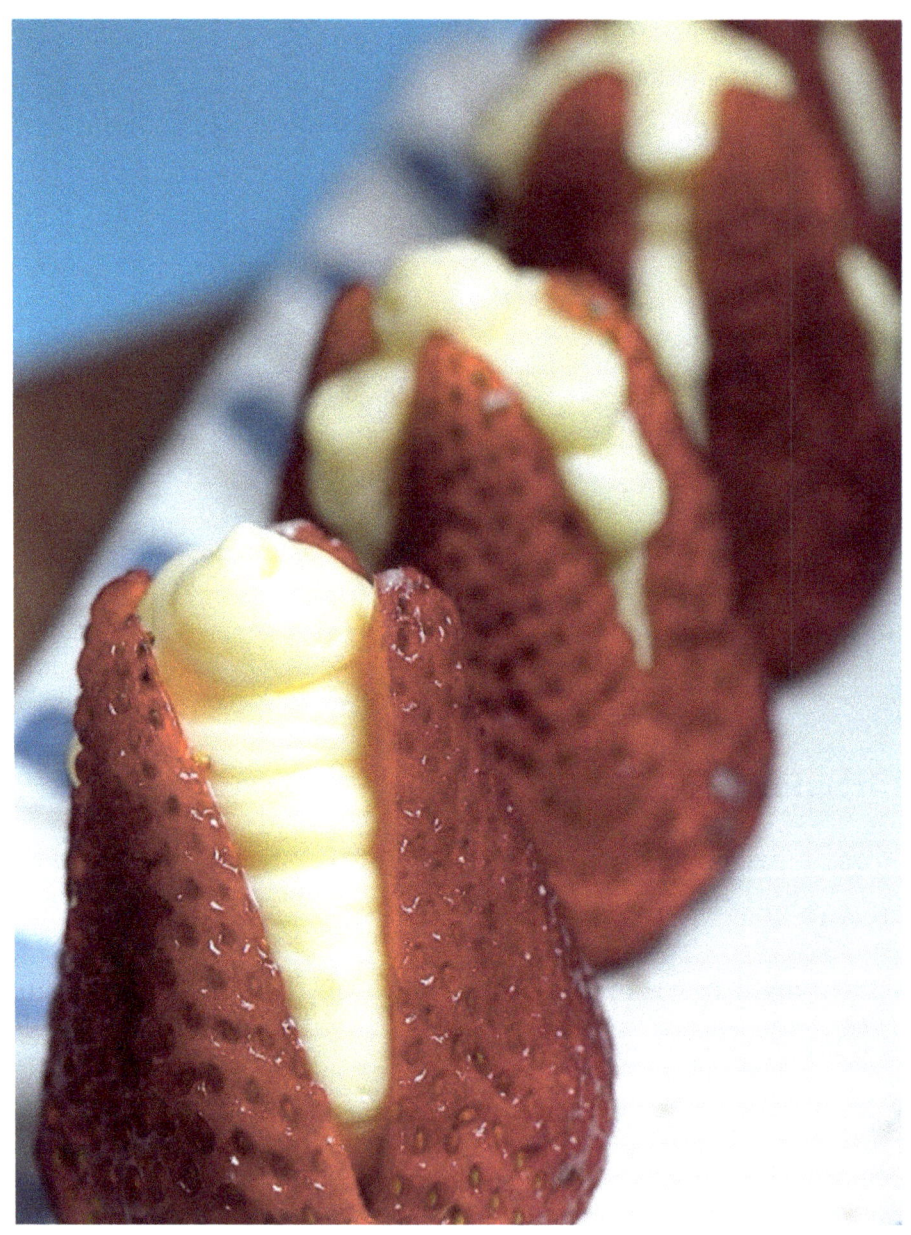

Tahini String Beans

Preparation Time: 15-30 minutes | Cooking Time: 10 minutes | Servings: 4

Ingredients:

• 1 tbsp sesame oil

• 1 cup string beans, trimmed

• Salt to taste

• 2 tbsp pure tahini

• 2 tbsp coarsely chopped mint leaves

• ¼ tsp red chili flakes for topping

Directions:

• Pour the string beans into a medium safe microwave dish, sprinkle with 1 tbsp of water, and steam in the microwave until softened, 1 minute.

• Heat the sesame oil in a large skillet and toss in the string beans until well coated in the butter.

• Season with salt and mix in the tahini and mint leaves. Cook for 1 to 2 minutes and turn the heat off.

• Plate the string beans and serve.

Nutrition:

Calories 79 kcal | Fats 4. 3g | Carbs 9. 5g | Protein 1. 27g

Black Beans Burger

Preparation Time: 15 minutes | Cooking Time: 5 minutes | Servings: 5

Ingredients:

• 1 cup black beans, cooked

• 2 tablespoons bread crumbs

• 1 teaspoon salt

• 1/4 cup sweet corn, cooked

• 1 teaspoon turmeric

• 1 tablespoon fresh parsley, chopped

• 1/2 yellow sweet pepper, chopped

• 1/2 cup of water

Directions:

• Mash the black beans until you get puree and combine them with salt, sweet corn, turmeric, parsley, and sweet pepper.

• Mix it up carefully with the help of a spoon.

• Add breadcrumbs and stir again.

• Pour water into the Pressure pot bowl and insert the steamer rack.

• Make the burgers from the black bean mixture and freeze them for 30 minutes.

• Then wrap every burger in the foil and place it on the steamer rack.

• Close the lid and cook on Manual mode (High pressure) for 5 minutes.

• Then allow natural pressure release for 5 minutes.

• Remove the foil from the burgers and transfer it to the plate. Garnish burgers with lettuce leaves if desired.

Nutrition:

Calories: 155 | Fat: 0.9 | Fiber: 6.5 | Carbs: 28.8 | Protein: 9.2

Mushroom Burger

Preparation Time: 10 minutes | Cooking Time: 14 minutes | Servings: 4

Ingredients:

- 2 cups mushrooms, chopped
- 1 onion, diced
- 1/2 cup silken tofu
- 1/2 teaspoon salt
- 1/2 teaspoon chili flakes
- 1 tablespoon dried parsley
- 1 teaspoon dried dill
- 3 tablespoon flax meal
- 1/2 teaspoon olive oil

Directions:

- Put mushrooms in the blender and grind.

• Then transfer the vegetables to the Pressure pot together with onion, and olive oil. Stir gently and close the lid. Cook Ingredients: on Sauté mode for 10 minutes.

• Meanwhile, mash silken tofu until you get a puree. Mix it up with salt, chili flakes, dried parsley, and dried dill. Add flax meal and pulse for 10 seconds.

• When the mushroom mixture is cooked transfer it to a bowl and combine it with the silken tofu.

• Stir well.

• Make the burgers.

• Line the Pressure pot pan with baking paper and place burgers on it.

• Close the lid and meal for 4 minutes on High. Then use quick pressure release.

• Chill the burgers to room temperature before serving.

Nutrition:

Calories: 47 | Fat: 2.6 | Fiber: 2.5 | Carbs: 5.4 | Protein: 2.6

Seitan Burgers

Preparation Time: 10 minutes | Cooking Time: 2 minutes |
Servings: 1

Ingredients:

• 1 burger bun

• 1 teaspoon mustard

• 1 teaspoon soy sauce

• 1 seitan steak

• 1 teaspoon onion powder

• 1 teaspoon olive oil

• 1 tablespoon apple cider vinegar

Directions:

• Make the sauce for seitan steak: mix up together soy sauce,
onion powder, olive oil, and apple cider vinegar.

• Brush seitan steak with sauce from each side and place in the
Pressure pot.

• Close the lid and cook on Manual mode (High pressure) for 2 minutes (quick pressure release).

• Meanwhile, cut the burger bun into halves and spread with mustard.

• Place seitan steak on the one half of the burger bun and cover with the second one.

Nutrition:

Calories: 303 | Fat: 8.8 | Fiber: 2.8 | Carbs: 24.9 | Protein: 26.8

Maple Roasted Squash

Preparation Time: 15-30 minutes | Cooking Time: 40 minutes | Servings: 4

Ingredients:

• 1 large butternut squash, deseeded and cubed

• 2 tbsp olive oil

• 4 garlic cloves, minced

• ¼ cup pure maple syrup

• Salt and black pepper to taste

• 1 tsp red chili flakes

• 1 tsp coriander seeds

• Preheat the oven to 375 F.

• In a medium bowl, toss the squash with the olive oil, garlic, maple syrup, salt, black pepper,red chili flakes, and coriander seeds.

• Spread the mixture on a baking sheet and roast in the oven for 25 to 30 minutes or until the potatoes soften and golden brown.

• Remove from the oven, plate, and serve warm.

Nutrition:

Calories 126 kcal | Fats 7. 1g | Carbs 15. 6g | Protein 1. 1g

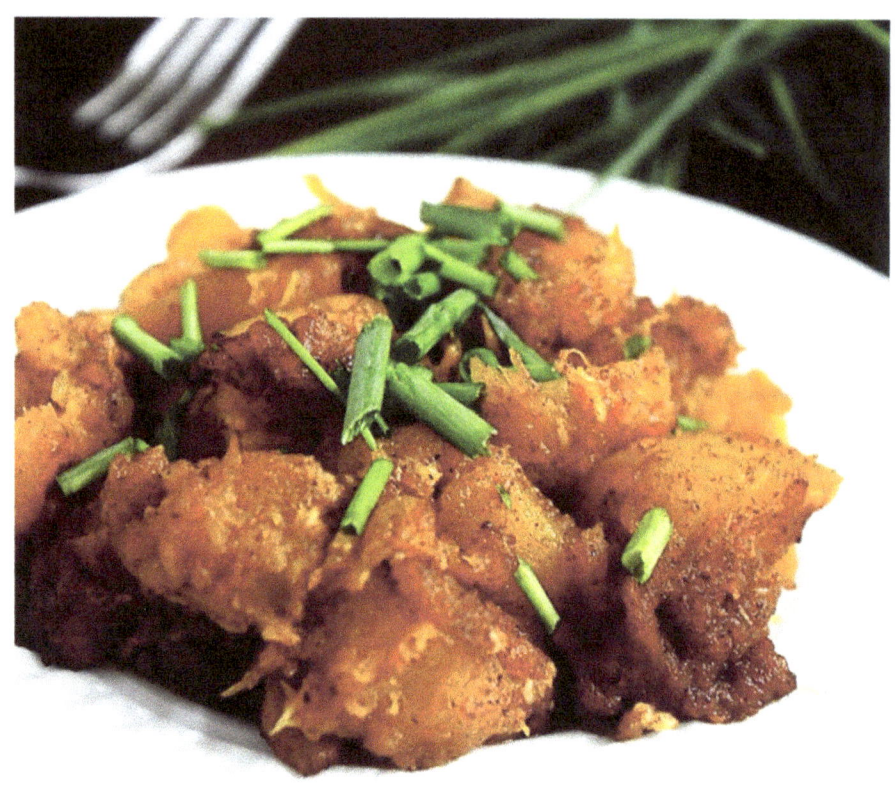

Carrot and Red Onion Sauté

Preparation Time: 15-30 minutes | Cooking Time: 20 minutes | Servings: 4

Ingredients:

• 2 beets, peeled and cut into wedges

• 3 small carrots, cut crosswise

• 2 tbsp plant butter

• 1 medium red onion, cut into wedges

• ½ tsp dried oregano

• 1/8 tsp salt

Directions:

• Steam the beets and carrots in a medium safe microwave bowl until softened, 6 minutes.

• Meanwhile, melt the butter in a large skillet and sauté the onion until softened, 3 minutes. Stir in the carrots, beets, oregano, and salt. Mix well and cook for 5 minutes. Dish the food into serving bowls and serve warm.

Nutrition:

Calories 95 kcal | Fats 6g | Carbs 10. 2g | Protein 1. 4g

Avocado Tomato Bruschetta

Preparation Time: 10 minutes | Cooking Time: 0 minute | Servings: 4

Ingredients:

- 3 slices of whole-grain bread

- 6 chopped cherry tomatoes

- ½ of sliced avocado

- ½ teaspoon minced garlic

- ½ teaspoon ground black pepper

- 2 tablespoons chopped basil

- ½ teaspoon of sea salt

- 1 teaspoon balsamic vinegar

Directions:

• Place tomatoes in a bowl, and then stir in vinegar until mixed. Top bread slices with avocado slices, then top evenly with tomato mixture, garlic, and basil, and season with salt and black pepper.

• Serve straight away

Nutrition:

• Calories: 131 Cal | Fat: 7.3 g | Carbs: 15 g | Protein: 2.8 g | Fiber: 3.2 g

Thai Snack Mix

Preparation Time: 15 minutes | Cooking Time: 90 minutes | Servings: 4

Ingredients:

- 5 cups mixed nuts
- 1 cup chopped dried pineapple
- 1 cup pumpkin seed
- 1 teaspoon garlic powder
- 1 teaspoon onion powder
- 2 teaspoons paprika
- 1 teaspoon of sea salt
- 1/4 cup coconut sugar
- 1/2 teaspoon red chili powder
- 1/2 teaspoon ground black pepper
- 1 tablespoon red pepper flakes
- 1/2 tablespoon red curry powder
- 2 tablespoons soy sauce

• 2 tablespoons coconut oil

Directions:

• Switch on the slow cooker, add all the ingredients in it except for dried pineapple and red pepper flakes, stir until combined, and cook for 90 minutes at a high heat setting, stirring every 30 minutes.

• When done, spread the nut mixture on a baking sheet lined with parchment paper and let it cool.

• Then spread dried pineapple on top, sprinkle with red pepper flakes and serve.

Nutrition:

Calories: 230 Cal | Fat: 17.5 g | Carbs: 11.5 g | Protein: 6.5 g | Fiber: 2 g

Zucchini Fritters

Preparation Time: 10 minutes | Cooking Time: 6 minutes | Servings: 12

Ingredients:

• 1/2 cup quinoa flour

• 3 1/2 cups shredded zucchini

• 1/2 cup chopped scallions

• 1/3 teaspoon ground black pepper

• 1 teaspoon salt

• 2 tablespoons coconut oil

• 2 flax eggs

Directions:

• Squeeze moisture from the zucchini by wrapping it in a cheesecloth and then transfer it to a bowl.

• Add remaining ingredients, except for oil, stir until combined, and then shape the mixture into twelve patties.

• Take a skillet pan, place it over medium-high heat, add oil and when hot, add patties and cook for 3 minutes per side until brown.

• Serve the patties with your favorite vegan sauce.

Nutrition:

Calories: 37 Cal | Fat: 1 g | Carbs: 4 g | Protein: 2 g | Fiber: 1 g

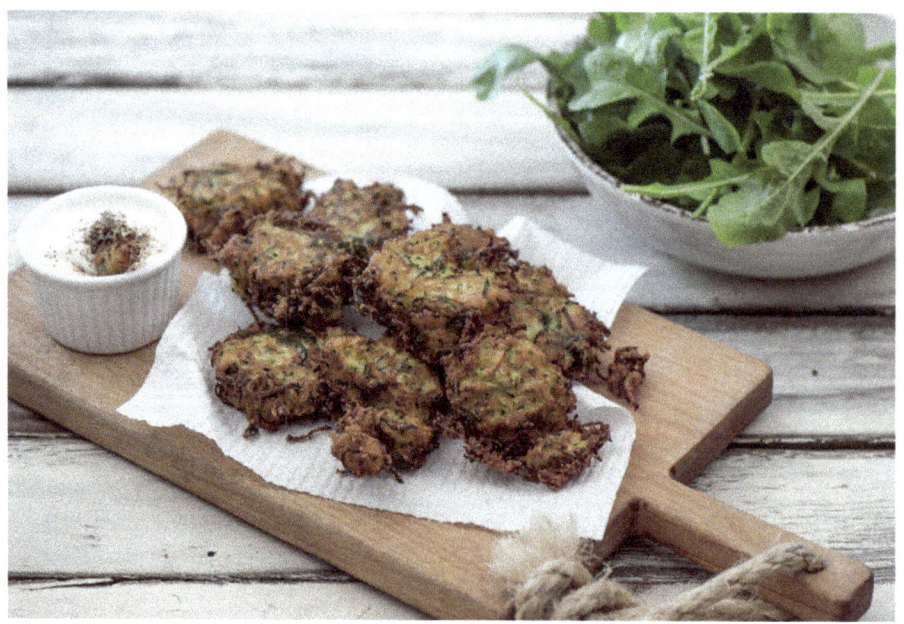

Zucchini Chips

Preparation Time: 10 minutes | Cooking Time: 120 minutes | Servings: 4

Ingredients:

• 1 large zucchini, thinly sliced

• 1 teaspoon salt

• 2 tablespoons olive oil

Directions:

• Pat dry zucchini slices and then spread them in an even layer on a baking sheet lined with parchment sheet.

• Whisk together salt and oil, brush this mixture over zucchini slices on both sides and then bake for 2 hours or more until brown and crispy.

• When done, let the chips cool for 10 minutes and then serve straight away.

Nutrition:

Calories: 54 Cal | Fat: 5 g | Carbs: 1 g | Protein: 0 g

Rosemary Beet Chips

Preparation Time: 10 minutes | Cooking Time: 20 minutes | Servings: 3

Ingredients:

- 3 large beets, scrubbed, thinly sliced

- 1/8 teaspoon ground black pepper

- ¼ teaspoon of sea salt

- 3 sprigs of rosemary, leaves chopped

- 4 tablespoons olive oil

Directions:

• Spread beet slices in a single layer between two large baking sheets, brush the slices with oil, then season with spices and rosemary, toss until well coated, and bake for 20 minutes at 375 degrees F until crispy, turning halfway.

• When done, let the chips cool for 10 minutes and then serve.

Nutrition:

Calories: 79 Cal | Fat: 4.7 g | Carbs: 8.6 g | Protein: 1.5 g | Fiber: 2.5 g

Quinoa Broccoli Tots

Preparation Time: 10 minutes | Cooking Time: 20 minutes | Servings: 16

Ingredients:

• 2 tablespoons quinoa flour

• 2 cups steamed and chopped broccoli florets

• 1/2 cup nutritional yeast

• 1 teaspoon garlic powder

• 1 teaspoon miso paste

• 2 flax eggs

• 2 tablespoons hummus

Directions:

• Place all the ingredients in a bowl, stir until well combined, and then shape the mixture into sixteen small balls.

• Arrange the balls on a baking sheet lined with parchment paper, spray with oil and bake at 400 degrees F for 20 minutes until brown, turning halfway.

- When done, let the tots cool for 10 minutes and then serve straight away.

Nutrition:

Calories: 19 Cal | Fat: 0 g | Carbs: 2 g | Protein: 1 g | Fiber: 0.5 g

Spicy Roasted Chickpeas

Preparation Time: 10 minutes | Cooking Time: 20 minutes | Servings: 6

Ingredients:

• 30 ounces cooked chickpeas

• ½ teaspoon salt

• 2 teaspoons mustard powder

• ½ teaspoon cayenne pepper

• 2 tablespoons olive oil

Directions:

• Place all the ingredients in a bowl and stir until well coated and then spread the chickpeas in an even layer on a baking sheet greased with oil.

• Bake the chickpeas for 20 minutes at 400 degrees F until golden brown and crispy and then serve straight away.

Nutrition:

Calories: 187.1 Cal | Fat: 7.4 g | Carbs: 24.2 g | Protein: 7.3 g |
Fiber: 6.3 g

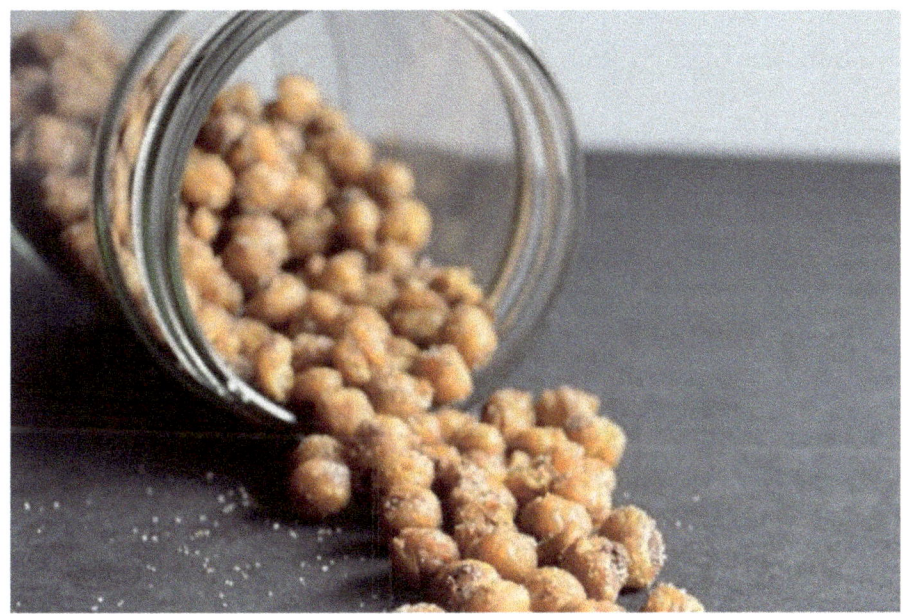

Nacho Kale Chips

Preparation Time: 10 minutes | Cooking Time: 14 hours | Servings: 10

Ingredients:

- 2 bunches of curly kale

- 2 cups cashews, soaked, drained

- 1/2 cup chopped red bell pepper

- 1 teaspoon garlic powder

- 1 teaspoon salt

- 2 tablespoons red chili powder

- 1/2 teaspoon smoked paprika

- 1/2 cup nutritional yeast

- 1 teaspoon cayenne

- 3 tablespoons lemon juice

- 3/4 cup water

Directions:

• Place all the ingredients except for kale in a food processor and pulse for 2 minutes until smooth.

• Place kale in a large bowl, pour in the blended mixture, mix until coated, and dehydrate for 14 hours at 120 degrees F until crispy.

• If a dehydrator is not available, spread kale between two baking sheets and bake for 90 minutes at 225 degrees F until crispy, flipping halfway.

• When done, let chips cool for 15 minutes and then serve.

Nutrition:

Calories: 191 Cal | Fat: 12 g | Carbs: 16 g | Protein: 9 g | Fiber: 2 g

Roasted Brussels Sprouts With Cranberries

Preparation Time: 15-30 minutes | Cooking Time: 50 minutes | Servings: 4

Ingredients:

• 1 pound Brussels sprouts, halved

• 3 tbsp olive oil

• Salt and black pepper to taste

• 1 medium white onion, chopped

• ½ cup dried cranberries

• 1 lemon, juiced

• 1 tbsp chopped fresh basil

Directions:

• Preheat the oven to 425 F.

• Spread the Brussels sprouts on a roasting sheet, drizzle with olive oil, and season with salt and black pepper.

• Mix the seasoning onto the vegetables and roast in the oven until light brown and tender, 20 to 25 minutes.

• Transfer the Brussels sprouts to a large salad bowl and mix in the onion, cranberries, lemon juice, and basil. Serve immediately.

Nutrition:

Calories 144 kcal | Fats 10. 4g | Carbs 12. 7g | Protein 2. 1g

Roasted Garlic Asparagus with Dijon Mustard

Preparation Time: 15-30 minutes | Cooking Time: 35 minutes | Servings: 4

Ingredients:

• 2 tbsp plant butter

• 1 lb asparagus, hard part trimmed

• 2 garlic cloves, minced

• 1 tsp Dijon mustard

• 1 tbsp freshly squeezed lemon juice

Directions:

• Melt the butter in a large skillet and sauté the asparagus until softened with some crunch, 7 minutes. Mix in the garlic and cook until fragrant, 30 seconds.

• Meanwhile, in a small bowl, quickly whisk the mustard, lemon juice and pour the mixture over the asparagus. Cook for 2 minutes and plate the asparagus. Serve warm.

Nutrition:

Calories 77 | Fats 6g | Carbs 5. 2g | Protein 2. 7g

Tofu Zucchini Kabobs

Preparation Time: 15-30 minutes | Cooking Time: 10 minutes | Servings: 4

Ingredients:

• 1 (14 oz) block extra-firm tofu, pressed and cut into 1-inch cubes

• 1 medium zucchini, cut into 2-inch rounds

• 1 tbsp olive oil

• 2 tbsp freshly squeezed lemon juice

• 1 tsp smoked paprika

• 1 tsp cumin powder

• 1 tsp garlic powder

Directions:

• Preheat a grill to medium heat.

• Meanwhile, thread the tofu and zucchini alternately on the wooden skewers.

• In a small bowl, whisk the olive oil, lemon juice, paprika, cumin powder, and garlic powder.

Brush the skewers all around with the mixture and place them on the grill grate.

• Cook on both sides until golden brown, 5 minutes. Serve afterward.

Nutrition:

Calories 147 | Fats 10. 3g | Carbs 5g | Protein 11. 9g

Chili Toasted Nuts

Preparation Time: 15-30 minutes | Cooking Time: 35 minutes | Servings: 4

Ingredients:

• 1 cup mixed nuts

• 1 tbsp plant butter, melted

• ¼ tsp hot sauce

• ¼ tsp garlic powder

• ¼ tsp onion powder

Directions:

• Preheat the oven to 350 F and line a baking sheet with baking paper.

• In a medium bowl, mix the nuts, butter, hot sauce, garlic powder, and onion powder. Spread the mixture on the baking sheet and toast in the oven for 10 minutes.

• Remove the sheet, allow complete cooling, and serve.

Nutrition:

Calories 267 | Fats 28. 3g | Carbs 4. 9g | Protein 2. 7g

Tangy Cabbage Stir-Fry

Preparation Time: 15-30 minutes | Cooking Time: 15 minutes | Servings: 4

Ingredients:

• 2 tbsp soy sauce

• 1 tbsp toasted sesame oil

• 1 tbsp hot sauce

• ½ tbsp pure date sugar

• ½ tbsp olive oil

• 1 head green cabbage, shredded

• 2 carrots, julienned

• 3 green onions, thinly sliced

• 2 garlic cloves, minced

• 1 tbsp fresh grated ginger

• Salt and black pepper to taste

• 1 tbsp sesame seeds

Directions:

• In a small bowl, mix the soy sauce, sesame oil, hot sauce, and date sugar.

• Heat the olive oil in a large skillet and sauté the cabbage, carrots, green onion, garlic, and

ginger until softened, 5 minutes.

• Mix in the prepared sauce and toss well. Cook for 1 to 2 minutes. Dish the food and garnish with the sesame seeds.

Nutrition:

Calories 126 kcal | Fats 8. 2g | Carbs 12. 6g | Protein 2. 4g

Marinated Mushrooms

Preparation Time: 10 minutes | Cooking Time: 7 minutes | Servings: 6

Ingredients:

- 12 ounces small button mushrooms

- 1 teaspoon minced garlic

- 1/4 teaspoon dried thyme

- 1/2 teaspoon sea salt

- 1/2 teaspoon dried basil

- 1/2 teaspoon red pepper flakes

- 1/4 teaspoon dried oregano

- 1/2 teaspoon maple syrup

- 1/4 cup apple cider vinegar

- 1/4 cup and 1 teaspoon olive oil

- 2 tablespoons chopped parsley

Directions:

• Take a skillet pan, place it over medium-high heat, add 1 teaspoon oil and when hot, add mushrooms and cook for 5 minutes until golden brown.

• Meanwhile, prepare the marinade and for this, place the remaining ingredients in a bowl and whisk until combined.

• When mushrooms have cooked, transfer them into the bowl of marinade and toss until well coated.

• Serve straight away

Nutrition:

• Calories: 103 Cal | Fat: 9 g | Carbs: 2 g | Protein: 1 g

Hummus Quesadillas

Preparation Time: 5 minutes | Cooking Time: 15 minutes | Servings: 1

Ingredients:

• 1 tortilla, whole wheat

• 1/4 cup diced roasted red peppers

• 1 cup baby spinach

• 1/3 teaspoon minced garlic

• ¼ teaspoon salt

• ¼ teaspoon ground black pepper

• 1/4 teaspoon olive oil

• 1/4 cup hummus

• Oil as needed

Directions:

• Place a large pan over medium heat, add oil and when hot, add red peppers and garlic, season with salt and black pepper, and cook for 3 minutes until sauté.

• Then stir in spinach, cook for 1 minute, remove the pan from heat and transfer the mixture to a bowl.

• Prepare quesadilla and for this, spread hummus on one-half of the tortilla, then spread spinach mixture on it, cover the filling with the other half of the tortilla and cook in a pan for 3 minutes per side until browned.

• When done, cut the quesadilla into wedges and serve.

Nutrition:

Calories: 187 Cal | Fat: 9 g | Carbs: 16.3 g | Protein: 10.4 g | Fiber: 0 g

Peanut Butter Blossom Biscuits

Preparation Time: 15-30 minutes | Cooking Time: 15 minutes + 1-hour chilling | Servings: 4

Ingredients:

• 1 tbsp flax seed powder + 3 tbsp water

• 1 cup pure date sugar + more for dusting

• ½ cup unsalted butter softened

• ½ cup creamy peanut butter

• 1 large egg, at room temperature

• 1 tsp vanilla extract

• 1 ¾ cup whole-wheat flour

• 1 tsp baking soda

• ¼ tsp salt

• ¼ cup unsweetened chocolate chips

Directions:

• In a small bowl, mix the flax seed powder with water and allow thickening for 5 minutes to make the flax egg.

• In a medium bowl using an electric mixer, whisk the date sugar, plant butter, and peanut butter until light and fluffy.

• Mix in the flax egg and vanilla until well combined. Add the flour, baking soda, salt, and whisk well again.

• Fold in the chocolate chips, cover the bowl with a plastic wrap, and refrigerate for 1 hour. After, preheat the oven to 375 F and line a baking sheet with parchment paper.

• Use a cookie sheet to scoop mounds of the batter onto the sheet with 1-inch intervals. Bake in the oven for 9 to 10 minutes or until golden brown and slightly cracked on top.

• Remove the cookies from the oven, cool for 3 minutes, roll in some date sugar, and serve.

Nutrition:

Calories 839 | Fats 52. 5g | Carbs 77. 9g | Protein 21. 1g

Black Bean and Corn Quesadillas

Preparation Time: 15 minutes | Cooking Time: 30 minutes | Servings: 4

Ingredients:

- For the Black Beans and Corn:

- 1/2 of a medium white onion, peeled, chopped

- 1/2 cup cooked black beans

- 1/2 cup cooked corn kernels

- 1 teaspoon minced garlic

- ½ of jalapeno, deseeded, diced

- 1/2 teaspoon salt

- 1 teaspoon red chili powder

- 1 teaspoon cumin

- 1 tablespoon olive oil

- For the Quesadillas:

- 4 large corn tortillas

- 4 green onions, chopped

- ½ cup vegan nacho cheese sauce

- ½ cup chopped cilantro

- 1 large tomato, diced

- Salsa as needed for dipping

Directions:

- Prepare beans and for this, take a frying pan, place it over medium-high heat, add oil, and when hot, add onion, jalapeno, and garlic and cook for 3 minutes.

- Then add remaining ingredients, stir until mixed and cook for 2 minutes until hot.

- Take a large skillet pan, place over medium heat, place the tortilla in it and cook for 1 minute until toasted, and then flip it.

- Spread some of the cheese sauce on one half of the top, spread with bean mixture, top with cilantro, onion, and tomato, and then fold the filling with the other side of the tortilla.

- Pat down the tortilla, cook it for 2 minutes, then carefully flip it, continue cooking for 2 minutes until hot, and then slide to a plate.

- Cook remaining quesadilla in the same manner, then cut them into wedges and serve.

Nutrition:

Calories: 251 Cal | Fat: 9.5 g | Carbs: 30.6 g | Protein: 15.6 g | Fiber: 12.1 g

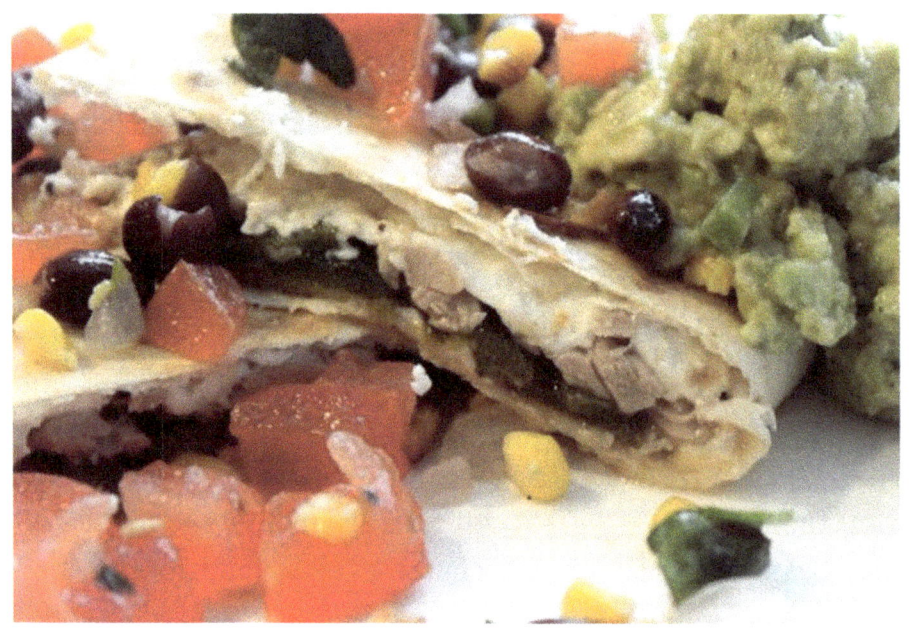

Oven-Dried Grapes

Preparation Time: 5 minutes | Cooking Time: 4 hours | Servings: 4

Ingredients:

• 3 large bunches of grapes, seedless

• Olive oil as needed for greasing

Directions:

• Spread grapes into two greased baking sheets and bake for 4 hours at 225 degrees F until semi-dried.

• When done, let the grape cool completely and then serve.

Nutrition:

Calories: 299 Cal | Fat: 1 g| Carbs: 79 g | Protein: 3.1 g | Fiber: 3.7 g

Stuffed Peppers

Preparation Time: 25 minutes | Cooking Time: 30-120 minutes | Servings: 5

Ingredients:

• 5 bell peppers, seeds removed

• 1 medium-sized onion, peeled and finely chopped

• 7 oz button mushrooms, sliced

• 4 garlic cloves, peeled and crushed

• 4 tbsp of extra-virgin olive oil

• 1 tsp of salt

• ¼ tsp of freshly ground black pepper

• ¼ cup of rice

• ½ tbsp. of cayenne pepper

Directions:

• Use package instructions to pre-cook the rice, or simply place ¼ cup of rice in 1 cup of water and bring it to a boil. Cook for 10 minutes.

• With the cooker's lid off, heat two tablespoons of olive oil and place the onion and crushed garlic in the stainless steel insert. Press ―Saute‖ and stir-fry until translucent and add mushrooms, salt, pepper, and cayenne pepper.

• Mix well and continue to cook until the water evaporates. Remove from the heat and combine with rice.

• Using a wooden spoon, combine the ingredients, and add the remaining olive oil.

• Use the mixture to stuff the pepper and gently transfer them to your Pressure pot.

• Securely lock the lid and press the ―Manual‖ button. Set the timer for 10 minutes and adjust the steam release handle. Cook on high pressure.

• When done, press the ―Cancel‖ button and release the steam naturally.

• Enjoy!

Nutrition:

Calories:680 | Total Fat:71.8g | Saturated Fat:20.9g | Total Carbs:10g | Dietary Fiber:7g | Sugar:2g | Protein:3g | Sodium:525mg

Quorn Sausage Frittata

Preparation Time: 10 minutes | Cooking Time: 33 minutes | Servings: 4

Ingredients:

- 12 whole eggs

- 1 cup plain unsweetened yogurt

- Salt and ground black pepper to taste

- 1 tbsp butter

- 1 celery stalk, chopped

- 12 oz Quorn sausages

- ¼ cup shredded cheddar cheese

Directions:

- Preheat the oven to 350 F.

- In a medium bowl, whisk the eggs, plain yogurt, salt, and black pepper.

• Melt the butter in a large (safe oven skillet over medium heat. Sauté the celery until soft, 5 minutes. Transfer the celery into a plate and set aside.

• Add the Quorn sausages to the skillet and cook until brown with frequent stirring to break the lumps that form for about 8 minutes.

• Flatten the Quorn sausage in the bottom of the skillet using the spoon, scatter the celery on top, pour the egg mixture all over, and sprinkle with the cheddar cheese.

• Put the skillet in the oven and bake until the eggs are set and cheese melts for about 20 minutes.

• Remove the skillet, slice the frittata, and serve warm with kale salad.

Nutrition:

Calories:293 | Total Fat:27.9g | Saturated Fat:2.9g | Total Carbs:11g | Dietary Fiber:4g | Sugar:2g | Protein:5g | Sodium:20mg

Brownie Energy Bites

Preparation Time: 1 hour and 10 minutes | Cooking Time: 0 minute | Servings: 2

Ingredients:

- 1/2 cup walnuts

- 1 cup Medjool dates, chopped

- 1/2 cup almonds

- 1/8 teaspoon salt

- 1/2 cup shredded coconut flakes

- 1/3 cup and 2 teaspoons cocoa powder, unsweetened

Directions:

• Place almonds and walnuts in a food processor and pulse for 3 minutes until the dough starts to come together.

• Add remaining ingredients, reserving ¼ cup of coconut, and pulse for 2 minutes until incorporated.

• Shape the mixture into balls, roll them in remaining coconut until coated, and refrigerate for 1 hour.

• Serve straight away

Nutrition:

Calories: 174.6 Cal | Fat: 8.1 g | Carbs: 25.5 g | Protein: 4.1 g | Fiber: 4.4 g

Strawberry Coconut Ice Cream

Preparation Time: 5 minutes | Cooking Time: 0 minute | Servings: 4

Ingredients:

• 4 cups frozen strawberries

• 1 vanilla bean, seeded

• 28 ounces coconut cream

• 1/2 cup maple syrup

Directions:

• Place cream in a food processor and pulse for 1 minute until soft peaks come together.

• Then tip the cream in a bowl, add remaining ingredients in the blender and blend until a thick mixture comes together.

• Add the mixture into the cream, fold until combined, and then transfer ice cream into a freezer-safe bowl and freeze for 4 hours until firm, whisking every 20 minutes after 1 hour. • Serve straight away.

Nutrition:

Calories: 100 Cal | Fat: 100 g | Carbs: 100 g | Protein: 100 g | Fiber: 100 g

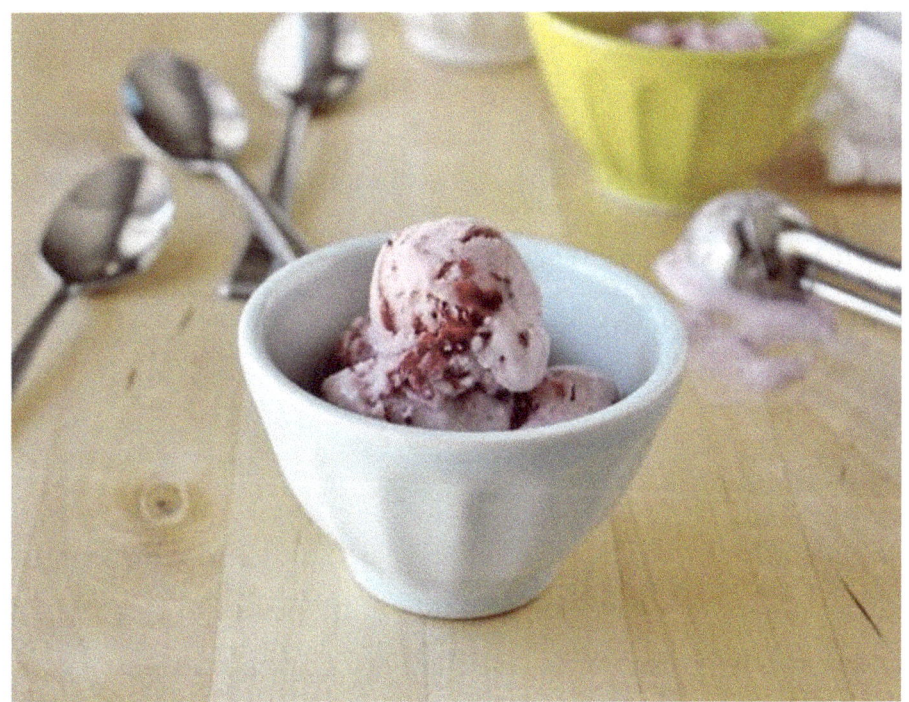

Salted Caramel Chocolate Cups

Preparation Time: 5 minutes | Cooking Time: 2 minutes | Servings: 12

Ingredients:

- ¼ teaspoon sea salt granules

- 1 cup dark chocolate chips, unsweetened

- 2 teaspoons coconut oil

- 6 tablespoons caramel sauce

Directions:

• Take a heatproof bowl, add chocolate chips and oil, stir until mixed, then microwave for 1 minute until melted, stir chocolate and continue heating in the microwave for 30 seconds.

• Take twelve mini muffin tins, line them with muffin liners, spoon a little bit of chocolate mixture into the tins, spread the chocolate in the bottom and along the sides, and freeze for 10 minutes until set.

• Then fill each cup with ½ tablespoon of caramel sauce, cover with remaining chocolate and freeze for another 2salto minutes until set.

• When ready to eat, peel off liner from the cup, sprinkle with sauce, and serve.

Nutrition:

Calories: 80 Cal | Fat: 5 g | Carbs: 10 g | Protein: 1 g | Fiber: 0.5 g

Chocolate Peanut Butter Energy Bites

Preparation Time: 1 hour and 5 minutes | Cooking Time: 0 minute | Servings: 4

Ingredients:

- 1/2 cup oats, old-fashioned
- 1/3 cup cocoa powder, unsweetened
- 1 cup dates, chopped
- 1/2 cup shredded coconut flakes, unsweetened
- 1/2 cup peanut butter

Directions:

• Place oats in a food processor along with dates and pulse for 1 minute until the paste starts to come together.

• Then add remaining ingredients, and blend until incorporated and a very thick mixture comes together.

• Shape the mixture into balls, refrigerate for 1 hour until set and then serve.

Nutrition:

Calories: 88.6 Cal | Fat: 5 g | Carbs: 10 g | Protein: 2.3 g | Fiber: 1.6 g

Mango Coconut Cheesecake

Preparation Time: 4 hours and 10 minutes | Cooking Time: 0 minute | Servings: 4

Ingredients:

For the Crust:

• 1 cup macadamia nuts

• 1 cup dates, pitted, soaked in hot water for 10 minutes

For the Filling:

• 2 cups cashews, soaked in warm water for 10 minutes

• 1/2 cup and 1 tablespoon maple syrup

• 1/3 cup and 2 tablespoons coconut oil

• 1/4 cup lemon juice

• 1/2 cup and 2 tablespoons coconut milk, unsweetened, chilled

For the Topping:

• 1 cup fresh mango slices

Directions:

• Prepare the crust, and for this, place nuts in a food processor and process until mixture resembles crumbs.

• Drain the dates, add them to the food processor and blend for 2 minutes until a thick mixture comes together.

• Take a 4-inch cheesecake pan, place date mixture in it, spread and press evenly, and set aside.

• Prepare the filling and for this, place all its ingredients in a food processor and blend for 3 minutes until smooth.

• Pour the filling into the crust, spread evenly, and then freeze for 4 hours until set. • Top the cake with mango slices and then serve.

Nutrition:

Calories: 200 Cal | Fat: 11 g | Carbs: 22.5 g | Protein: 2 g | Fiber: 1 g

Rainbow Fruit Salad

Preparation Time: 10 minutes | Cooking Time: 0 minute | Servings: 4

Ingredients:

For the Fruit Salad:

- 1 pound strawberries, hulled, sliced

- 1 cup kiwis, halved, cubed

- 1 1/4 cups blueberries

- 1 1/3 cups blackberries

- 1 cup pineapple chunks

For the Maple Lime Dressing:

- 2 teaspoons lime zest

- 1/4 cup maple syrup

- 1 tablespoon lime juice

Directions:

• Prepare the salad, and for this, take a bowl, place all its ingredients and toss until mixed.

• Prepare the dressing, and for this, take a small bowl, place all its ingredients and whisk well.

• Drizzle the dressing over salad, toss until coated, and serve.

Nutrition:

Calories: 88.1 Cal | Fat: 0.4 g | Carbs: 22.6 g | Protein: 1.1 g | Fiber: 2.8 g

Cookie Dough Bites

Preparation Time: 4 hours and 10 minutes | Cooking Time: 0 minute | Servings: 18

Ingredients:

• 15 ounces cooked chickpeas

• 1/3 cup vegan chocolate chips

• 1/3 cup and 2 tablespoons peanut butter

• 8 Medjool dates pitted

• 1 teaspoon vanilla extract, unsweetened

• 2 tablespoons maple syrup

• 1 1/2 tablespoons almond milk, unsweetened

Directions:

• Place chickpeas in a food processor along with dates, butter, and vanilla and then process for 2 minutes until smooth.

• Add remaining ingredients, except for chocolate chips, and then pulse for 1 minute until blended and dough comes together.

- Add chocolate chips, stir until just mixed, then shape the mixture into 18 balls and refrigerate for 4 hours until firm.

- Serve straight away

Nutrition:

Calories: 200 Cal | Fat: 9 g | Carbs: 26 g | Protein: 1 g | Fiber: 0 g

Chocolate & Almond Butter Barks

Preparation Time: 15-30 minutes | Cooking Time: 35 minutes | Servings: 4

Ingredients:

• 1/3 cup coconut oil, melted

• ¼ cup almond butter, melted

• 2 tbsp unsweetened coconut flakes.

• 1 tsp pure maple syrup

• A pinch of ground rock salt

• ¼ cup unsweetened cocoa nibs

Directions:

• Line a baking tray with baking paper and set aside.

• In a medium bowl, mix the coconut oil, almond butter, coconut flakes, maple syrup, and then fold in the rock salt and cocoa nibs.

• Pour and spread the mixture on the baking sheet, chill in the refrigerator for 20 minutes or until firm.

• Remove the dessert, break it into shards, and enjoy it immediately.

• Preserve extras in the refrigerator.

Nutrition:

Calories 279 | Fats 28. 1g | Carbs 8. 6g | Protein 4. 4g

Mini Berry Tarts

Preparation Time: 15-30 minutes | Cooking Time: 35 minutes + 1-hour chilling | Servings: 4

Ingredients:

- For the pie crust:

- 4 tbsp flax seed powder + 12 tbsp water

- 1/3 cup whole-wheat flour + more for dusting

- ½ tsp salt

- ¼ cup plant butter, cold and crumbled

- 3 tbsp pure malt syrup

- 1 ½ tsp vanilla extract

- For the filling:

- 6 oz cashew cream

- 6 tbsp pure date sugar

- ¾ tsp vanilla extract

- 1 cup mixed frozen berries

Directions:

• Preheat the oven to 350 F and grease a mini pie pan with cooking spray.

• In a medium bowl, mix the flax seed powder with water and allow soaking for 5 minutes.

• In a large bowl, combine the flour and salt. Add the butter and using an electric hand mixer, whisk until crumbly. Pour in the flax egg, malt syrup, vanilla, and mix until smooth dough forms.

• Flatten the dough on a flat surface, cover with plastic wrap, and refrigerate for 1 hour.

• After, lightly dust a working surface with some flour, remove the dough onto the surface, and using a rolling pin, flatten the dough into a 1-inch diameter circle,

• Use a large cookie cutter, cut out rounds of the dough and fit into the pie pans. Use a knife to trim the edges of the pan. Lay a parchment paper on the dough cups, pour on some baking beans, and bake in the oven until golden brown, 15 to 20 minutes.

• Remove the pans from the oven, pour out the baking beans, and allow cooling.

• In a medium bowl, mix the cashew cream, date sugar, and vanilla extract.

• Divide the mixture into the tart cups and top with berries. Serve immediately.

Nutrition:

Calories 545 | Fats 33. 5g | Carbs 53. 6g | Protein 10. 6g

Mixed Nut Chocolate Fudge

Preparation Time: 15-30 minutes | Cooking Time: 2 hours 10 minutes | Servings: 4

Ingredients:

• 3 cups unsweetened chocolate chips

• ¼ cup thick coconut milk

• 1 ½ tsp vanilla extract

• A pinch salt

• 1 cup chopped mixed nuts

Directions:

• Line a 9-inch square pan with baking paper and set aside.

• Melt the chocolate chips, coconut milk, and vanilla in a medium pot over low heat.

• Mix in the salt and nuts until well distributed and pour the mixture into the square pan.

• Refrigerate for at least 2 hours.

• Remove from the fridge, cut into squares, and serve.

Nutrition:

Calories 907 | Fats 31. 5g | Carbs 152. 1g | Protein 7. 7g

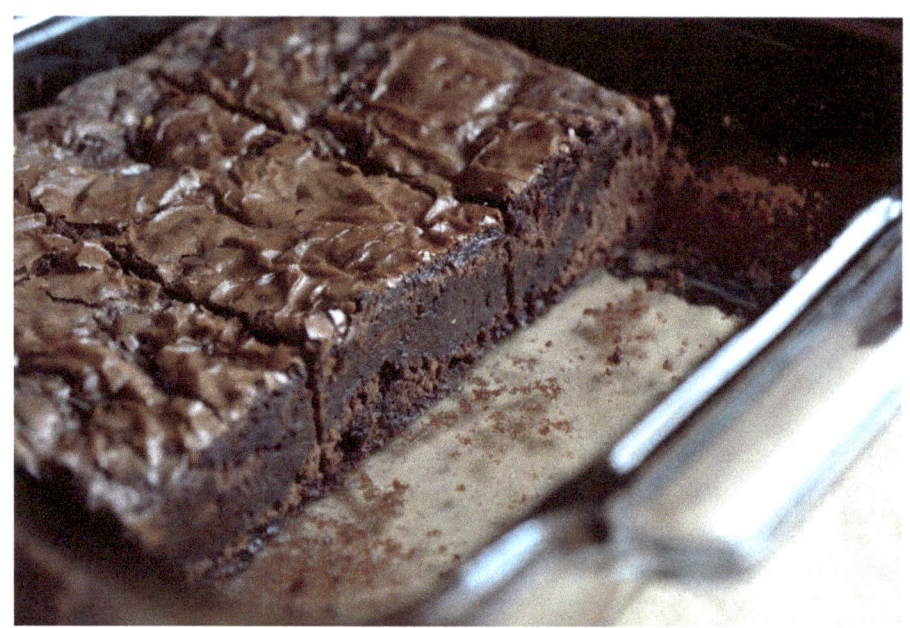

Date Cake Slices

Preparation Time: 15-30 minutes | Cooking Time: 1 hour 20 minutes | Servings: 4

Ingredients:

- ½ cup cold plant butter, cut in pieces, plus extra for greasing

- 1 tbsp flax seed powder + 3 tbsp water

- ½ cup whole-wheat flour, plus extra for dusting

- ¼ cup chopped pecans and walnuts

- 1 tsp baking powder

- 1 tsp baking soda

- 1 tsp cinnamon powder

- 1 tsp salt

- 1/3 cup water

- 1/3 cup pitted dates, chopped

- ½ cup pure date sugar

- 1 tsp vanilla extract

- ¼ cup pure date syrup for drizzling.

Directions:

• Preheat the oven to 350 F and lightly grease a round baking dish with some plant butter.

• In a small bowl, mix the flax seed powder with water and allow thickening for 5 minutes to make the flax egg.

• In a food processor, add the flour, nuts, baking powder, baking soda, cinnamon powder, and salt. Blend until well combined.

• Add the water, dates, date sugar, and vanilla. Process until smooth with tiny pieces of dates evident.

• Pour the batter into the baking dish and bake in the oven for 1 hour and 10 minutes or until a toothpick inserted comes out clean. Remove the dish from the oven, invert the cake onto a

serving platter to cool, drizzle with the date syrup, slice, and serve.

Nutrition:

Calories 850 | Fats 61. 2g | Carbs 65. 7g | Protein 12. 8g

Chocolate Mousse Cake

Preparation Time: 15-30 minutes | Cooking Time: 40 minutes + 6 hours 30 minutes chilling | Servings: 4

Ingredients:

• 2/3 cup toasted almond flour

• ¼ cup unsalted plant butter, melted

• 2 cups unsweetened chocolate bars, broken into pieces

• 2 ½ cups coconut cream

• Fresh raspberries or strawberries for topping

Directions:

• Lightly grease a 9-inch springform pan with some plant butter and set aside.

• Mix the almond flour and plant butter in a medium bowl and pour the mixture into the springform pan. Use the spoon to spread and press the mixture into the bottom of the pan. Place in the refrigerator to firm for 30 minutes.

• Meanwhile, pour the chocolate into a safe microwave bowl and melt for 1 minute stirring every 30 seconds.

• Remove from the microwave and mix in the coconut cream and maple syrup.

• Remove the cake pan from the oven, pour the chocolate mixture on top making sure to shake the pan and even the layer. Chill further for 4 to 6 hours.

• Take out the pan from the fridge, release the cake and garnish with the raspberries or strawberries.

• Slice and serve.

Nutrition:

Calories 608 | Fats 60. 5g | Carbs 19. 8g | Protein 6. 3g

Apple Raspberry Cobbler

Preparation Time: 15-30 minutes | Cooking Time: 50 minutes | Servings: 4

Ingredients:

- 3 apples, peeled, cored, and chopped

- 2 tbsp pure date sugar

- 1 cup fresh raspberries

- 2 tbsp unsalted plant butter

- ½ cup whole-wheat flour

- 1 cup toasted rolled oats

- 2 tbsp pure date sugar

- 1 tsp cinnamon powder

Directions:

- Preheat the oven to 350 F and grease a baking dish with some plant butter.

- Add the apples, date sugar, and 3 tbsp of water to a medium pot. Cook over low heat until the date sugar melts and then, mix in the raspberries. Cook until the fruits soften, 10 minutes.

• Pour and spread the fruit mixture into the baking dish and set aside.

• In a blender, add the plant butter, flour, oats, date sugar, and cinnamon powder. Pulse a few times until crumbly.

• Spoon and spread the mixture on the fruit mix until evenly layered.

• Bake in the oven for 25 to 30 minutes or until golden brown on top.

• Remove the dessert, allow cooling for 2 minutes, and serve.

Nutrition:

Calories 539 | Fats 12g | Carbs 105. 7g | Protein 8. 2g

White Chocolate Pudding

Preparation Time: 15-30 minutes | Cooking Time: 4 hours 20 minutes | Servings: 4

Ingredients:

• 3 tbsp flaxseed + 9 tbsp water

• 3 tbsp cornstarch

• ¼ tbsp salt

• 1 cup cashew cream

• 2 ½ cups almond milk

• ½ pure date sugar

• 1 tbsp vanilla caviar

• 6 oz unsweetened white chocolate chips

• Whipped coconut cream for topping

• Sliced bananas and raspberries for topping

Directions:

• In a small bowl, mix the flax seed powder with water and allow thickening for 5 minutes to make the flax egg.

• In a large bowl, whisk the cornstarch and salt, and then slowly mix in the cashew cream until smooth. Whisk in the flax egg until well combined.

• Pour the almond milk into a pot and whisk in the date sugar. Cook over medium heat while frequently stirring until the sugar dissolves. Reduce the heat to low and simmer until steamy and bubbly around the edges.

• Pour half of the almond milk mixture into the flax egg mix, whisk well and pour this mixture into the remaining milk content in the pot. Whisk continuously until well combined.

• Bring the new mixture to a boil over medium heat while still frequently stirring and scraping all the corners of the pot, 2 minutes.

• Turn the heat off, stir in the vanilla caviar, then the white chocolate chips until melted. Spoon the mixture into a bowl, allow cooling for 2 minutes, cover with plastic wraps making sure to press the plastic onto the surface of the pudding, and refrigerate for 4 hours.

• Remove the pudding from the fridge, take off the plastic wrap, and whip for about a minute.

• Spoon the dessert into serving cups, swirl some coconut whipping cream on top, and top with the bananas and raspberries. Enjoy immediately.

Nutrition:

Calories 654 | Fats 47. 9g | Carbs 52. 1g | Protein 7. 3g

Cardamom Coconut Fat Bombs

Preparation Time: 5minutes | Cooking Time: 2minutes | Servings: 6

Ingredients:

- ½ cup unsweetened grated coconut

- 3 oz. unsalted butter, room temperature

- ¼ tsp green cardamom powder

- ½ tsp vanilla extract

- ¼ tsp cinnamon powder

Directions:

• Pour the grated coconut into a skillet and roast until lightly brown. Set aside to cool. • In a bowl, combine the butter, half of the coconut, cardamom, vanilla, and cinnamon. • Use your hands to form bite-size balls from the mixture and roll each in the remaining coconut.

• Refrigerate the balls until ready to serve.

Nutrition:

Calories: 687 | Total Fat: 54.5g | Saturated Fat: 27.4 g | Total Carbs: 9g | Dietary Fiber: 2g | Sugar: 4g | Protein: 38g | Sodium: 883 mg

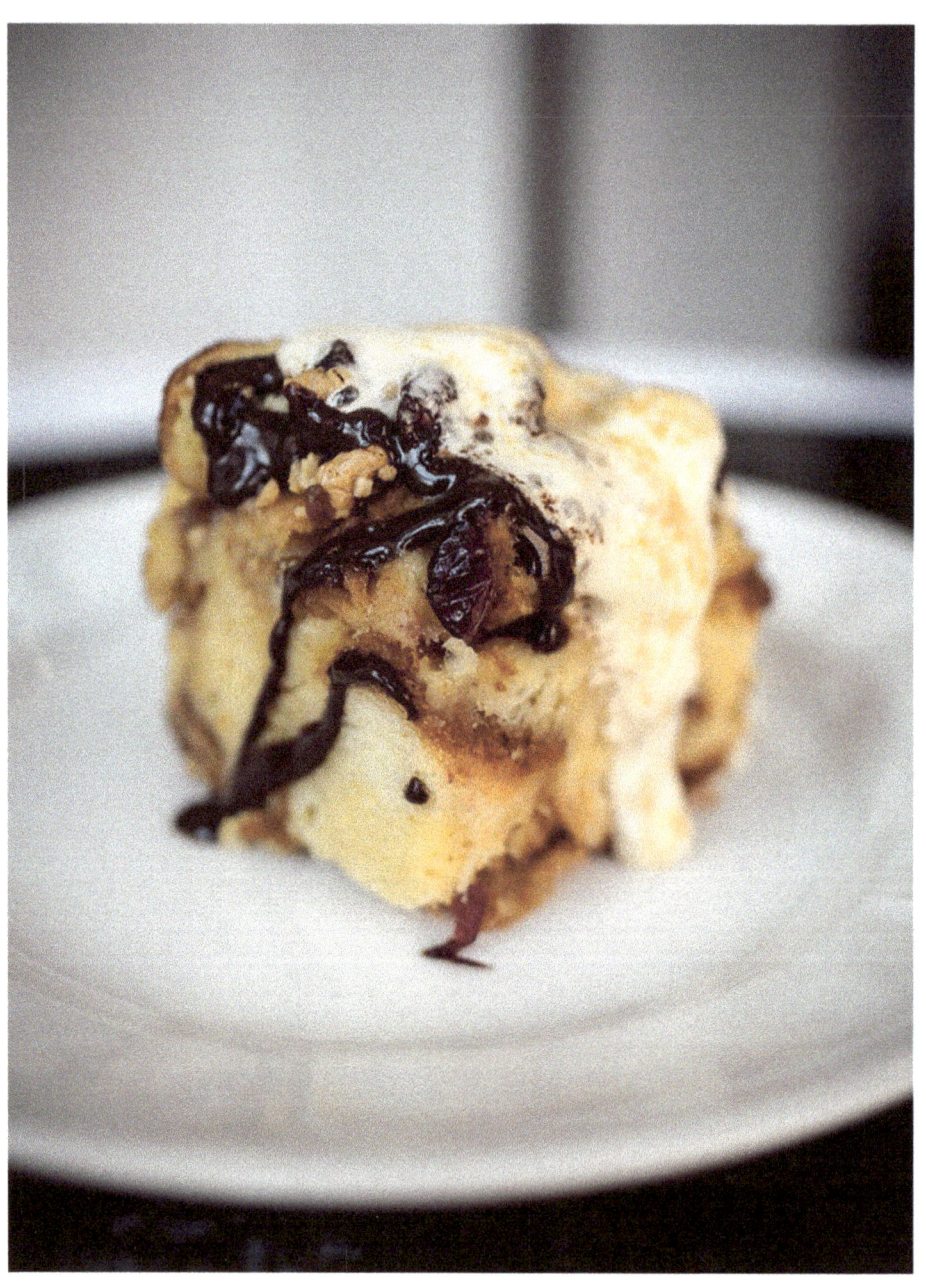

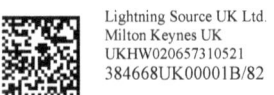

Lightning Source UK Ltd.
Milton Keynes UK
UKHW020657310521
384668UK00001B/82